Journal Of An
Alzheimer's Caregiver

Journal Of An Alzheimer's Caregiver

Winifred E. Johnson

authorHOUSE®

AuthorHouse™
1663 Liberty Drive
Bloomington, IN 47403
www.authorhouse.com
Phone: 1-800-839-8640

Published by AuthorHouse   04/20/2012

ISBN: 978-1-4685-7640-5 (sc)
ISBN: 978-1-4685-7639-9 (e)

Dedicated to my loving husband Bob who first encouraged me to put my thoughts in print.

Many thanks to my daughters: Patricia Headman Phyllis Johnson, Pamella Mahlum, and my friend Jean Schwartz who helped me edit my book

There probably is not one senior who thinks of Alzheimer's and wonders if it will strike him or her. They see friends succumb to the ravaging disease, and frankly, it frightens them. I am one of those seniors.

My husband, Bob, was diagnosed with Vascular Dementia, I asked the doctor what was the difference between this Alzheimer's and Vascular Dementia. "Nothing, the result is the same". he said. "However there will be highs and lows in the durations of this disease".

The next step I took was to look up everything I could about Alzheimer's, to find out what it was all about. Here are some feelings about Alzheimer's: It is death by a thousand subtractions, it is the long good-bye, like a slow deepening fog, it robs by degrees the person we love. (Nancy Reagon) Five million people have it and it lasts about eight years or less.

Bob, my husband, was known to have this disease for the last six years of his life. However, I was concerned about this disease for quite a few years before that. I learned about long term memory, that lasts forever. Short term memory takes about a month to form a long term memory. With Alzheimer's early on you lose your ability to form any new memories. I sure found that this is true. With this disease you start to lose one after another of your systems. The first to go is the memory, the thinking part of the brain. Along with this is confusion about everything, poor judgment and personality changes. Next you lose muscle control, for walking and standing, bladder control and eventually all body functions. Then on to regulatory functions eating and breathing.

People have asked me when I first noticed that anything was wrong. That is a hard one to answer because as Carl Sandburg said in a poem "The fog comes on little cat feet". Gradually everything in your life changes. It is really later on that you can go back, especially if you have a journal (which I have) and see what was going on related to dementia and how it has effected your loved ones life and your own.

My husband Bob was an intellectual. He had a Doctorate degree in Education and also was an ordained minister. He was pastor of a little church in Hainesport New Jersey for several years. Then established, and was the administrator, at Maranatha Children's Home in Fairbanks, Alaska. Both of us worked together to serve the Alaskan Indian and Eskimo children We were there as missionaries under the Conservative Baptist Home Mission Society. We left there after serving for twelve years. It was hard to leave.

We moved to Bellingham, Washington where Bob attended Washington State College. He received his BS in education there. We moved to Silverdale, Washington where he taught junior high students.

After two years our Conservative Baptist Home Mission Society called us back to the mission field in Cottonwood, Arizona. Here Bob became the administrator at the Navaho Bible School. Again we worked together teaching the Navaho people the Bible. It was while living there that he worked on his Doctorate in Education. We were there for four years. During the four years I got my BA in education.

We moved to Bothell, Washington where he completed his Doctorate in Education. During our time in Bothell he taught at Seattle Pacific University. His classes were to teach young people how to be teachers. This was his specialty. He enjoyed working with his students and helping them to grow. He was well liked by all of his students. I was one of his students while working on my Master's Degree.

Again we moved this time to Sequim, Washington where Bob was the principal at an elementary school. I was a teacher in a Elementary School in Port Angeles. We both retired in1980 after a few years of being a principal and me a teacher.

We both were involved in making pottery. After retiring we made it a business and sold various items that we made.

Retirement didn't agree with him at all so he sought a volunteering job at the Master's College in Newhall, Calif. We sold our home in

Sequim and moved to Newhall. Once more we both worked together with the students at the college. He was well liked at this college also and did similar work to that of Seattle Pacific University. Eventually this became a paying job. He also worked wih students at Azusa College in Azusa, Calif.

We moved from the college community to Hemet, Calif., where we bought a mobile home. Bob commuted to the colleges. This was pretty hard on him. Traffic was very heavy from Hemet to Newhall. so we moved back to Newhall where he continued to to teach. We bought a Condo there.

It was in his teaching that I first noticed his decline. In 1988 he was teaching at the Master's College. Everything was going along fine and then he would come home and seem agitated. This was because he was finding it hard to find the words that he wanted to use in the classroom. At the time I was not thinking of Alzheimer's, I was just concerned for him. Also at this time retirement seemed like a good choice. He did retire from both colleges.

After selling our two homes, eventually we moved to Camano Island, Washington. It was there that I began to see some changes in Bob that were unusual for him. He was having a great deal of difficulty balancing the check book. He said to leave it up to the bank. Gradually I took over balancing the check book and paying the bills. This was new to me but I took this in my stride.

He enjoyed reading very much and preferred that to listening and watching TV. Gradually, however, he started to lose interest in the newspaper. He stopped reading books, I think because it was too hard to follow the story. He liked me to tell him about the books I was reading. It was difficult for him to follow a story line, so he lost his interest in TV movie's. He did enjoy working with a golden retriever to train her for a handicapped person, this was bringing some meaning to his life. He enjoyed it very much and did a good work with the dog. This lasted for a year.

We enjoyed our life on Camano. We had a nice home and beautiful gardens. The deer would come into the yard and eat from our fruit trees. We joined a fine church there. I was active in the woman's group and felt like I was contributing to the church and to the Lord. Bob taught an adult Sunday School class. We also had a ministry of visiting those people who were sick and house bound.

After a few years Bob expressed a desire to move again. I delayed as long as I could. It was with much regret I finally gave in. Bob's request was that we move closer to the hospital in Mount Vernon, Washington. He was very active in buying a new home.

It was a good move because our home on Camano Island was on the side of a big hill, and now our home was on a nice level street where and we could get out walking. He did fine with this, however, he began having problems with his balance. Quite a few times he fell on the side walk or even on the road. Every time he fell it was always on his head, he couldn't remember to put out his hands to protect himself. I was beginning to feel very wary for him going out on walks by himself, so I would go with him when he walked the dog.

In talking to the doctor about this problem he did not feel that Bob was doing all that bad, He just urged him to walk to get some strength.

About now I was beginning to wonder about Alzheimer's, he was having lots of headaches and loss of balance. So I took him to a neurologist who evaluated him and said he was fine, no problems. He had me take Bob and have a MRI on his head. It was discovered that his basal nerve cell clusters had a twisted winding course in his brain that was very unusual. It was thought that this could be causing his headaches and loss of balance. At the time the doctor said this had nothing to do with Alzheimer's. However, I couldn't help but wonder.

It was this loss of balance that caused him to fall in our small bathroom, and hit his head on the wall. Bob was just pitiful, he was laying in a heap and I was unable to help him, he was just too heavy. He was throwing up blood. I called a neighbor and he helped Bob out of the bathroom, but advised me to call 911 right away. Which I did. They checked him over and took him to the hospital. At that time they did not label him as having Alzheimer's. He was there a few days and then I opted to have him in a nursing home until he was a little stronger. Bob had always said that he would like to go to a nursing home, so I did not feel bad about this move at all.

The nursing home in Mount Vernon was very nice, and he thoroughly enjoyed being there and having all the attention of everyone on him. I was glad he was getting the attention and I was grateful that they were giving him some physical therapy to help his balance.

After he came home from the nursing home we had nurses come in several times a week to check up on him and give me advice on how to handle things. He improved a lot but still had poor balance. When he got walking again, he fell down many times.

Some mornings I would wake up and wonder how I was going to cope with the day ahead. Will I be able to meet these new challenges in my life.

One week he refused to take his medicine, he said, "I'm in charge here I don't have to take it". We got through that one. However I felt like he was going backward in his health. I suggested that we try and get him some help. I took him to a psychologist but she was not much help. She just tried altering his medications and adding more depressant medication.

There was a nice gym in our town and Bob and I thought maybe that would help him to have better balance. That lasted about a month, then Bob was bored with that and did not want to make the effort to go.

After this he seemed to act different, as though everything was just too much effort to extend himself. He had been enjoying church, but now found excuses every Sunday for why he should not go to church. He was less talkative and seemed depressed at times. He seemed mixed up in his mind. For instance I was talking about President Clinton and he did not know who he was even after I told him he was our president.

Then there are other days when he seemed perfectly normal, knew what was going on and was interested in everything and seems quite happy.

Along came a day when we were in the restaurant eating and suddenly Bob said, "I feel like I am going backward". It seems he had been reading about a man like him who liked restaurants and he was diagnosed as manic depressive. Later the man killed himself. He asked me to look up about manic depressive people. He frightened me with this request. I asked the Lord to guide me on how to handle this.

Our daughter Pam lived about an hour and a half away from our home in Bothell, Washington and they had decided to move to Tacoma because of her husband Chuck's job. I suddenly felt very insecure myself, I wanted to be closer to family, especially with the way Bob seemed to be going. Frankly, I was afraid of being all alone in Mount Vernon with my children many miles away from us when Bob was in this condition.

We put our house up for sale and actually it sold very quickly, but we had to put some needed work into it. That was in the month of July 1999 and we drove down to Tacoma to look at homes in that month. My husband and I went together to look at all the possibilities. Finally we found one that he liked and signed the papers and bought it. It was not long after we bought the house and moved in that Bob started saying "I want to go home". He also denied ever signing any papers and said this was not our home. I was not really sure of where home was in his mind. This was not a one time happening, it happened every time we went out in the car, as well as times at the house.

The house was very adequate and I was liking it by the end of August. It is wonderful to be near family. All the members of our family came to visit us there. Right then all was well in our world.

Bob started having bad dreams and would wake up frightened. One time he was sure I had died and he didn't know what to do. I assured him I was his wife. At times he acted very remote like he didn't know what was going on.

By September I was having a lot of difficulty with the stress of every day living. Bob now had difficulty in dressing himself and it was a struggle for me to dress him. He was constantly tired and wanted to go back to bed a lot. I started to have trouble sleeping and some times a week would go by without a good nights sleep.

Eventually it became very hard to take care of Bob and I had to have a home care giver come in and bath him and help him shave and take care of his body. The man that came would take care of him and I could go out and do the family shopping for an hour. It was a real blessing to have the home health care people drop by to help me with the physical changes in my Bob.

He went through a period of wanting to expose his body to the world, and that was hard. I had to be on my guard and be ready to cover him up. I conducted a Bible Study group in my house and it was during these meetings that I had to be on the alert all the time.

One day I was preoccupied with cleaning the house and suddenly realized he was missing. I went outside and saw him walking down the street. He said he was going to the restaurant to get some doughnuts. It took a lot of convincing to have him turn around and come back to the house with me.

During all this time at home he was very difficult to feed. He was not pleased with anything I made. I lost all my confidence in cooking during this time. Even in shopping for food I felt lost as to what he would like to eat. For instance he loved doughnuts, so I bought some filled doughnuts that he really liked. When I served them to him he said he did not like that kind and wished I bought the sugar kind.

In January of 2000, Bob had to have surgery on his eye for retinal detachment. This disturbed him a lot, and he thought he was losing his sight. He began to seem very frail and I took him to the doctor. They discovered he was dehydrated and real weak. At my daughter and my suggestion he was put into the hospital for a check up. At this point his speech was slurred. The doctor there thought he had a mild stroke and his acids levels were way up. This doctor also suspected, for the first time, that Bob had Alzheimer's.

From the hospital he went to a nursing home. He was given physical therapy there to build up his strength. After a week of physical therapy Bob's speech became much better. I guess he began feeling somewhat better, in fact so much so that in the middle of the night he got up, dressed, packed up his stuff and went to the lobby to wait for his daughter to pick him up. Around the end of the month we brought him home.

At home he was still a handful, so we were fortunate to have a group of people work with him at home, physical therapists, speech therapists, physical care people. All this was a blessing to me, because he was so big, over 230 pounds and almost six feet tall. I was glad to have them help him physically. He would not exercise when they were not there.

By February 2000 he needed oxygen just to move around the house or for any activity. He began falling frequently. I bought him a walker to aid in moving around in the house, but he did not like to use it. This helped a good deal when he was willing to use it.

During the year we were in and out of the doctor's office. Bob had bronchitis and was getting weaker and weaker. I bought him a scooter so that he could get outside, but he only used it a couple of times.

Also during this month he fell and hurt his ribs. Fortunately they were not cracked, but Bob was uncomfortable.

We were fortunate to get a geriatic doctor who was willing to accept new patients. He was recommended to us by one of the nurses who came to visit him. He was a very good doctor.

By November the doctor took tests for Alzheimer's on Bob. He said Bob had vascular dementia and this overlaps to Alzhimer's, the outcome is just the same. He failed the tests and I was amazed at how hard it was for him to answer simple questions and to draw a clock and put the numbers on the face of the clock. I felt like crying. This was also the cut off date for Bob to stop driving. For which I was glad,

I already was doing most of the driving and did not feel safe when he drove.

Life went on, accepting the knowledge that my husband had vascular dementia. It was hard knowing that things would not be getting any better, but would instead get much worse. What I needed was courage, and I prayed for that.

At one of our doctor's visits he suggested that I read the book "36 Hour Day" by Nancy Maceand and Peter V. Rabins I did and read it all the way through. What an insight into Alzheimer's this is. The things it said would happen either did happen or had happened as the years went by. It also enlightened me as to what to expect in the future and also how to interpret the past.

For a while Bob was obsessed with sex, I found that this does happen in many people, so you learn to take it in your stride.

One day my very good friend Betty came for a visit, we had a very nice time. However during her visit my husband started to make an indecent proposal to her. I caught his drift in time to change the subject. Later Betty and I discussed his condition and she suggested that I invest in a lawyer to settle my affairs and consider a nursing home. Her mother had been going thru the same thing. That evening I discused the problem with him and he just changed the subject. The next morning when I greeted him he said "I just want a good meal and then I can die". I wondered if this had anything to do with of the conversation of the night before.

Also his moods would go way up really excited, about for instance, buying up all the houses surrounding us and becoming a real estate dealer along with his son. He would sound very rational in what he was saying except it would never be possible financially. I happened to call my son that day and Bob wanted to talk to him. He told our son to quit his job and go into partnership with him on a big real estate deal. Paul just agreed with him. Then the next day he would be down in a funk.

Another morning he woke up went to the living room and starting hollering for me. He told me he was sick and needed to go to a doctor or hospital at 2:30AM. I took his blood pressure and it was high. I calmed him down and fed him some food and coaxed him back to bed and soon he was off to sleep. Not me, I was too concerned.

Bob loved to eat out in restaurant's, but it was a real chore for me. First off he would be fussy where we ate, then couldn't make up his mind what to eat, and then when it came usually he took from one and half to two hours to eat.

Once more I was hiring a man to come in and take care of Bob's daily needs. He was very good and so helpful to Bob. At one day we had a woman substitute for the man, and she was clearly afraid of my husband. She was so grateful when I got home from shopping. There was Bob standing in the hallway with half of his clothes on, said he was looking for that woman. We decided never to have another woman come in and care for him.

I was still trying to get to church, I knew Bob would go back to bed after breakfast. So I went to church and the pastor preached on "The Valley of the Shadow of Death". That set me off, I had to leave the santuary and go to the restroom and cry. A friend came in to comfort me. I had to leave church for home.

Through the years as I write down each day's activities I felt that my computer is therapy for me. I wrote out my feelings and it sometimes releases the anger. Most nights I would wake up every hour or so to check up on Bob. On one of these nights I found Bob in the living room and he was hollering to me that he was cold. Turns out the thermostat was not working and it took me two hours to get it working again, but I did it. This was all new to me, Bob had been the one to take care of everything in the house.

One day I was having dizzy spells, so I laid down to rest. Bob came in and wanted me to start packing up just the pictures in the house because he felt they were the only things that really mattered in our house. He questioned me about if we had a car and if so lets get it packed and go. Just get out of here and get home.

In October of 2001 I took Bob to the doctor, it was such trouble getting him dressed and ready to go that by the time I got there I was exhausted. I made arrangements to see one of the other doctors to help me cope with all of this.

We had a sunny day in October and Bob took his walker and went out in the yard to get some sun. Later I looked out and he was laying with his bathrobe wide open and showing off his depends. There are young people in the area, and I was so afraid that they would see him. However he could not get out of his chair, so I got his scooter and through a lot of maneuvering finally got him in the house.

This same month I began loosing control of myself. Much to my own horror and his I shouted at him. I had never done that before in my life. This confused him more. When I talked to the doctor about this, she said you need to get away for a week by myself. Easier said than done when you are responsible for the man you love. At her suggestion I started taking Zoloft. She said I was way off the scale for stress and I needed some relief. She also cautioned me that Bob could become violent with me. That of course did not help to relieve my stress at all, but the Zoloft did.

Bob started roaming at night, one night he went outside, fortunately our little dog started barking and woke me up and I searched for him and found him not too far from home. He was walking as fast as he could with his walker. He said, "I'm looking for my supper". I convinced him to come on in and I would fix him a meal. Which I did. However from then on I had a chair under the handle of the outside door and a waste paper basket on top in case he started to move the chair. I figured the noise would wake me up.

The very next day Bob got up with a nice shirt and pants on and his hair all slicked back, all very unusual for him. So I told him, "You look very nice, are you going someplace special". He said "Yes, I need my violin because I am going out to visit a little old lady and I am going to play hymns for her on the violin". There was a time when he could have done this, he played a lot when he was a young man. As the day progressed his plans were forgotten.

There came a day when Bob felt wonderful, like a little boy. He looked down at his place mat and just could not get over how beautiful it was. It was the same place mat that we had been using for over a week. He wanted to call his brother and have him come and enjoy the place mat with him.

One night he woke me up at 3:30 AM. He said "Get right up and save yourself because we are getting gas in the house". He opened all the doors and windows to let the fresh air in, and put the fans on to move the gas. He was concerned for all the neighbors also and said they were going to die if they were not warned. The plan he had was to gather all of the people from all over into a large auditorium where they would be safe. I went around closing doors and windows and he sat in his chair lamenting that we would all die. I told him the Lord was going to take care of us, but this did not help his anguish. I finally got him comforted.

Later on in the day he again talked about packing up the pictures and leaving because this was not his home, he never signed any papers for it. The papers were signed by him, but he was not really with it when we moved here.

He kept telling me he was going to cry. I told him that was okay. He said no one cared if he cried, and I told him it was alright to cry if he wanted to. Then I prayed with him with the emphasis on him, this helped.

I was having more dizzy spells all the time, and I was becoming extremely tired. There were times when Bob was quite normal and talked like he used to. Other times he was extremely quiet.

At a foot doctor appointment Bob became obsessed with the idea that the doctor got a degree from college to trim toenails. While in the Doc's office he wanted to berate him for getting a degree for doing something that his Grandfather did in the bathtub when he was a child. I successfully shut him up before he said something that would embarrass us both.

At another doctor's appointment Bob got surly with the nurse saying he didn't want to be there. He didn't like it because the doctor talked rather fast and he could not hear what he was saying. Can't say as I might not feel the same way if I could not hear.

One afternoon Bob was really upset. He wanted to know where his father was. When I told him he died, he started to cry, just thinking he would never see his Dad again made him sad. He was in the mode, right then, that he had to take care of the whole family somehow. He would not even accept that his Mother had died because he knows he saw her within the last week. It took a while to comfort him in these situations.

In November Bob had it in his head that we would put our Dodge Caravan on a train with all of our things and go East on a trip. While there he wanted to go up to his Uncle Doug's farm and buy a place that is up on the hill. Then put some people in there to care for it. He also wanted to get someone to take care of the place here. I didn't know what was really in his mind but it sure was traveling.

Sometimes I felt like I couldn't handle things any more. I consantly had to go to the Lord for support during those days of utter confusion. Bob had begun to wet the bed, which made it hard each day.

On and off Pam, our daughter, and I looked at nursing homes. But now, finally I started to be serious about finding one. It was not a pleasant task for me, I had so many misgivings.

After breakfast one morning Bob wanted to talk, he needed to be straightened out. He could not understand how his brother Don had the same Mom as him. He again wanted to be straightened out where everyone lived. Actually as far as conversation goes he sounded normal but the thinking process was twisted. We talked for two hours, I don't know how far I got in straightening him out.

On November 8th I went to my first Alzheimer's meeting, it was all about what is being done for victims of Alzheimer's. It was a help for me to know of all the other people who are in the same boat as me. We all had different problems to meet with and yet similar.

The doctor sometime in November, I think, gave Bob medicine for erratic behavior, it was supposed to control his sexual urges. However it did not work for him.

There were times when Bob was so confused he could not find his way around the house to the bedroom or bathroom. I stayed close by him on those days.

One morning he woke up crying, I helped him get dressed and he felt a little better. I had to take the dog to be groomed that morning, so I had to leave him. When I got back he was agitated wanted to know where his dog was. Also, where was his wife Winifred was, he needed her. I explained to him who I was. For the rest of the day whenever I went out of the room I would tell him where I was going, this seemed to help

Soon after Thanksgiving Bob went through a period where he did not know who I was or where we were living. It was two days after Thanksgiving and Bob couldn't remember that day at all. He could not remember our son Paul being with us also.

After lunch that day Bob was telling me that he was the boss of all the railroads in the nation and that he would need some good help and wanted me to help him. I agreed to help him. Two days later he was telling me that he had a train right out the front door and we could go and pick up his brother Don and his wife Joyce.

He also thought he had a check for over a thousand dollars and wanted to go out and buy me some nice jewelry. Also he expected a lot of people to come and eat with us and thought they were very rude not to arrive.

Bob was still talking about trains at the end of November, and wanted me to take the train out shopping, he wanted to know how I felt about the train. His brother Don and wife came to visit, and Bob spent quite a bit of time talking to them about his train and invited them to bring up their grandson James to ride on the train.

On Bob's birthday, Dec 6, Pam brought some things over for him and we had a nice birthday party with just the two of us. We went out in the afternoon and I was going to shop but on the way I got a tight pain in my chest, then the pain went up in my jaw. I turned the car off the freeway and headed home. When I stopped the car I explained to Bob that I thought I was having a heart attack. He said, "Well go right ahead". I took my medicine at the house and rested for about a half hour. This was so different from the Bob I knew, to act this way.

Later on I asked him to get a can of soup. He really got upset he didn't know how to get a can of soup. I just wanted him to get it from the laundry room closet. So he put on his hat and said he was going out to look for his brother Don. I begged him not to go out, because if he did I would have to go out too and I felt very tired. Eventually I got him calmed down and I got the can of soup and fixed it for us.

One day I was doing some shopping and visited my doctor. When I got home Bob questioned me about being at the airport. It turns out that there was some trouble there and he was sure he had seen me there when he was watching the TV.

I drove us down to Cannon Beach, Oregon for a little break. My daughter in law called me and asked me to turn on the TV. When

I turned it on the reporters were commenting on the terrible trama going on in New York City. It was Sept. 11 2001. I commented on how terrible this was for our nation. Bob did not realize what was going on. He just looked at me and did not make any comment.

On December 9, 2001 Bob told me that he had cried all night because his wife had died. I assured him that I was his wife and I had not died. I served him breakfast and we just put on TV and enjoyed some good preaching. Then I put on a turkey to cook so that we could eat a late dinner. When he came to the table, he sat down and I served him. He looked at the food and said I don't think I can eat turkey and gravy. I told him that was okay and that I would fix him anything he wanted. Shortly after that he suddenly sort of threw himself back in his chair and his eyes rolled back into his head. I was screaming Bob, Bob can you hear me Bob. He did not respond. I wanted to take his pulse, but I was so nervous I could not even find a pulse in his neck. So I ran for the phone and called 911, the operator was asking me questions and all I could say was my husband needs help, help. My daughter Pam and her husband Chuck had called earlier and said they were coming over, and while I was on the 911 call they came in the door. Talk about timing it was just perfect. So they took over the calling. Pam tried to calm me down. Chuck kept looking after Bob. The medics were here very fast. They took care of Bob testing for vital signs, they also at Pam's insistence took my blood pressure. Mine was way up and I really do not know what Bob's was. They took him off to the St. Claire hospital. Chuck told me that even if Dad did go to heaven, he would be going to get a place ready for me, I thought that was so sweet.

Pam took care of the leftovers of the meal and I just sat there. We left about a half hour later to the hospital. They did the usual check up's and a CAT scan. We were there from around 4:30 to 8:15PM. They decided to keep Bob in the hospital over night. They tried to get our own Doctor Reginball but couldn't contact him. So we went home.

Chuck and Pam took me home and said to be sure to eat. Finally I ate the food that I had prepared earlier. Then went to bed very late. I ended the day with a prayer that God would take care of my Bob

It was a very poor night for me, and when I called the hospital at 3AM, it was not a very good night for Bob either. He was having trouble breathing and he was not comfortable. The doctor says it is possible that he just stopped breathing for that time yesterday. It certainly was terrible to go through. He also said that he had some fluid in one lung and they were wanting to take care of this so that he did not get pneumonia. So the doctor decided to keep him a few days until he felt that Bob was in good shape.

We thought that after this he should go to a nursing home for a while to see how he makes out before they let him come home or put him into a nursing facility permanently. This was a hard decision for me to make and I really needed the input from my doctor to know what he thinks and where would he suggest that Bob be taken.

Bob did not look good to me, he was having such a bad time breathing. I stayed with him for a while. This was really a scary time for me. The day went by like a blur, waiting for doctors and not getting any information. I was having a hard time thinking staight. They seemed to have no way of knowing what happened to Bob.

Pam and I planned to go to see nursing homes in the morning. Then go see Bob. Well the Doc called and said that he was ready to discharge him right away. That blew my mind because we were not ready and I told him so. He said he would wait until Thursday to release him. Since we would be taking him to a nursing home, I was concerned that this would be a good decision on my part.

Pam took me to a nursing home the next morning, but we did not have time to go through it because I wanted to get to see Bob as soon as possible. So we went to see him and I was so glad that we did, because he looked so much better. He was still having trouble swallowing, but I think that is improving. He recognized me, he said, "I'm glad the train let you off". Still thinking he owned the trains.

Pam and I spent a lot of time going to other nursing homes to evaluate them. This was a big decision to make for us. We visited several of them.

My next trip to the hospital Bob was very alert and that made me feel good. My friends at church had been keeping me in prayer and that meant a lot to me, it gave me comfort. I went to the Bible Study group and it was good to get away for a little while.

Pam took me back to the hospital after the meeting. Bob was asleep, but I took his hand anyway and he held on really tight. He woke up and told me he liked me holding his hand. He wanted me to get in bed with him and warm him up. They brought his supper while I was there and the nurse came to feed him. We left then and I was glad because I was very tired.

On December 13, 2001, Bob went into the nursing home. So I gathered some of his clothing and toiletries together in a suitcase. We were going to Heartwood Nursing Home and we will see how this goes for Bob.

Pam and I stayed with him and then we went to the office to fill in the paper work. Chuck, Pam's husband, came by from work and Bob was so glad to see him. Bob did not like it that I was not with him in the morning at the nurseing home.

What would really be strange is I thought that I would no longer be the one to make decisions for his health, the nursing home would be the ones. I wouldn't be the one to get the medicine and be sure that he takes it. I would not be conferring with the doctor. I felt that my usefulness had gone as far as my husband is concerned.

On my first visit to his room I looked around to think what might make him feel more at home. So I brought some pictures, a small TV and plants. He does not have much room to put things. He was sort of bound to a wheel chair. He can get up and down however. The people in physical therapy have him walk down the hall a little way, to keep up the strength in his legs. I decided to give him a ride and I pushed him all around the facility. After pushing him around I was plum exhausted. When Bob went to lunch, I looked in at him, he was using a weighted spoon and had difficulty eating still. He eats just a little bit of food. Then we left while he was eating.

Bob began trying to get out of bed unassisted again. I was afraid he would fall. He wanted me to gather everyone together and get off the train. I went along with it for a while. But then thought he really needs to know that he is in a nursing home. He was looking for Caroline (his mother).

I was going to stay until 4:10, figuring that I could get home before dark. I was just about deciding to go when the fire alarm went off. Scared me half to death. Then the door of the room closed and locked. After a bit a nurse came in to see if all was okay in the room and it was. I heard them talking about the fire engine. However they told me that nothing was wrong, it was just a rehearsal. Good to know they have practices.

Pam took me in for a visit in the morning and again in the afternoon. My son Paul and his wife Linda came from their home to visit Bob. Bob was telling us that his arm was bothering him. I thought it was from laying on it. He told Paul it was hurting. Paul thought it was from them lifting him.

Soon after Bob was in the nursing home his arm started swelling. I was quite concerned and told the staff so. Pam, Tolena, my granddaughter and I took Bob to a diagnostic center to try and find out what is wrong with his arm. It was difficult getting him in and out of the car, but it was worth it to find out what was wrong. We discovered later from the nurse that there was a blockage of the blood in his arm and that it was phlebitis. So the Doctor prescribed some medication to relieve the pain.

There came a point where the nurses were feeding him. Then one day he said, "I am feeding myself". I congradulated him and he was insulted and said, "I always have fed myself". Any activity made Bob tired, eating exhausts him, going to the bathroom exhausts him, he does best in bed actually, where of course he falls asleep.

The nursing home had special programs all year long, Christmas was a happy time in the dining room. Families of patients were invited to come and join in the fun. Santa Claus was there and each patient had their picture taken with him. They served a great meal Bob ate a small portion of this. This was all before the actual day of Christmas.

For Christmas Bob came home for the day. We had to thicken his liquids because he is having trouble swallowing. I was happy that he could be with us, but he was anxious to get back to his bed. These are tough days for Bob, because he really is not aware of what is happening to him.

The transit system bus came and picked Bob up. I spent the rest of the holiday at Pam & Chucks house, so I was not as lonely as I thought I would be.

After Christmas I had to decide whether to bring Bob home or not. I was encouraged by my family and the staff to let him stay there. This was difficult for me to do, I felt I was reneging on my wedding vows. Especially the part "Till Death do us part". I didn't want him to be there, I wanted him home. I knew I would miss just having his presence with me. Somehow there was something so final about making that decision. Finally I decided that he should stay there. No sooner had that decision been made, when I went back to see Bob, he was mad, he wanted to go home now. Immediately I began feeling guilty.

When New Years Eve came it was the first time since we were married that we did not pray the New Year in. But I did it by myself with the Lord at my side. The new year is going to be difficult I know but the Lord is going to take care of our needs and guide us in the right direction.

I started encouraging Bob to use his feet to move his wheel chair. Soon after that the nurses told me that he was going down the halls very fast. They were concerned for him and other residents.

One day the nurse called from the nursing home saying that Bob wanted to leave and go to China so he could get pretzels. She wanted me to bring him some, but I told her he could not eat them. Anyway I hurried to the home, stoped at Baskin Robins and got some ice cream for Bob. He was glad to get the ice cream, but he still wanted to go to China, just to have some Chinese food he said. I asked him if he was just kidding and he said yes. I talked to the nurse and she said he really was giving them a time he really wanted to get out the front door and was insistent about it. They had a hard job calming him down.

With the reality of Bob not coming home I was thinking of selling my house, which I hated to leave and getting an apartment that Chuck and Pam and the family would build on Pam's first floor. Chuck has some good ideas. I decided to go for that. Selling our home will be very hard for me. I would miss all that I had there, but I do know that much of what I had I do not really need. It was just the business of getting rid of things.

Have been looking into having someone come in to look after Bob, so that he could come to the apartment, to live. We would have liked someone to help me with him. However I discovered that this would not work. We could not afford it.

Bob was having hallucinations of seeing his mother, he thinks she is on the second floor. There is no second floor to the nursing home. Occasionally Bob seems to know me, I was so glad when that happened. Other times he does not know who I am at all. His short term memory is shot, couldn't remember from one hour to the next. He seems always tired and I asked the nurse if this was part of the dementia and she said yes. In order for him to get up it took two people to help him out of bed or into bed.

As time went on I learned to tell Bob this is what we are going to do, instead of asking him what he wanted to do. If I asked him he will answer with, "No". One time when I asked him "Who Loves you", he answered "My mother". Then I said, "Who else", and he said "No one". These kind of questions are useless, they only hurt your feelings.

I was talking to a social worker about this and she suggested that I make a list of my stresses and this is what I wrote.

External Stresses:

1. Caring for Bob even though he is in the Nursing Home.
2. Trying to figure out what is best for him.
3. Figuring out the financial end of living permanently in a Nursing Home.
4. Getting the information that will be needed for Medicaid.
5. Getting rid of some of my things in preparation for moving into Pam's house.
6. Making sure my Bible Study lesson is done.

Internal Stresses:

1. The agony of keeping Bob in a nursing home.
2. The agony of knowing he will never be coming home again.
3. The guilt of doing all this to him after all those years.
4. To be able to release the fact that MY BOB will never be the same again.
5. That I may show him love even when he does not show any back.
6. That I may do what the LORD wants me to do in my life as well as Bob's.
7. I am so tired, and I feel like I will be tired the rest of my life, I feel like I will never feel truly happy again as far as my worldly life is concerned, I need to rest in the strength of the Lord continually and sometimes I slip. PLEASE LORD keep me focused.

Bob had a roommate and he seemed like a nice man, but he is frequently called out "Jack The Ripper" and that sort of makes me a little frightened. In the four years he was at Heartwood he has had several roommates. One man was continually trying to fix things in the room, or being unhappy because of something that is going on. Another time he thought I was his wife. The only thing one can do is be kind and gentle with them, they are all in the same boat. I find that I am losing energy, and I too am very tired.

I read, "A Caregiver's Survival Guide", by Kay Marshall Strom. In the chapter dealing with loses. She said, "I think the worst loss of all was the loss of being two people who cared for and about each other. Gone were our shared interests. Gone were our dreams for the future. Gone were the stimulating conversations and thought-provoking discussions. Gone was my sense of security and safety. Gone was the husband I had known and loved. I read all that and thought that they were truly all gone.

Then the next chapter was titled, Finding the Blessing. I looked at that and cried, how can I find a blessing in this. What I found is that I have had more love and joy in my life than most people have had, because for one thing the Lord has let me live so long with Bob. I must think on those things rather than what could have been. Also I must remember that God has been so good to us through the years and that through all of this I have come into a closer relationship with God. I miss my Bob that I used to have and ask God to forgive me for putting him in a nursing home. I prayed that he will find some interest there that he could not find at home.

During January 2002 I had to make the final decision, would I bring Bob home and try to care for him, or would I have to go to Medicaid to keep Bob in the nursing home. Financially that decision was made for me, the people at Heartwood told me what the finances would amount to. I knew I could not handle that. I would have to use the government and I just hated to do that. Also I realized that I was not strong enough to care for him.

Bob had times of knowing me and talking to me and I would read him jokes and show him pictures that I thought he would enjoy. These happy times for us happened infrequently while he was living there.

One morning I woke up to a snowy world and the snow still falling. It was beautiful out I must admit. However I felt in the depths of despair. I wonder what had I done to Bob, how could I do that. I missed him so much even though he did not talk much to me I still missed him. I missed having him near me. I asked the Lord for comfort and assurance that all of this is alright in His eyes. O Lord I need you.

After Medicare took over he was moved to a new room and it was right by a schools playground, he enjoyed watching all of the children playing out in the yard. I think it reminded him of when he was a principal.

While I was with him these days I felt his anger, he would not recognize me, he seemed to want to shove me out of his life. That is the last thing I wanted.

I watched a movie that ended with a husband and a wife kissing and saying "I Love You". I burst out in tears, I don't ever expect to hear that again and I just can't believe it. How could life go down the drain so quickly. I was still in a depressed mood I couldn't seem to get out of this. Was I grieving, I didn't know. I just did not want to go and see Bob when he would not acknowledge that I was there or even look at me. This was a major depression for me to bear.

I would eat one meal a week with Bob. I would feed him his food soon after I started because he was too tired to lift his utensils. At times this would be a pleasant occasion where Bob would actually talk to me. As years rolled by he quit reacting and it was merely a time of feeding him and talking to him. I enjoyed being able to feed him this made me feel a little bit useful.

Once in a while when I came to see Bob he would have a great big grin of recognition. A couple of times he told me "I'm so glad you came". These were important times for me.

The doctor put Bob on Zoloft, he was in deep depression. The doctor said he just says, "What's the use of doing anything". I grieved because of that statement, it brought tears to my eyes right away and later many tears. I felt if only I could handle him I would have him home. He needed me and I needed him. If only he would take the trouble to try and stand, then we could plan on getting him out at least once a month, maybe more. I felt like he wasn't trying but in reality he had lost the ability to use his feet. Oh Heavenly Father help me to help him in some way.

I would bring his beloved dog Randy in to visit him. When I first brought him he was really happy. At later times he did not react to him at all.

I grieved for Bob in my heart. I prayed all the way to Heartwood that he would be receptive. I also tried very hard to turn this all over to the Lord and let him guide me in what I say to Bob, because I didn't know what to say. I would give lots of hugs and kisses. This truly had been the hardest time of my life. I tried to express this to Bob. I think he should know that I was not happy that he is there, that I really care.

On one of Bob's more coherent days he asked me, "What is up for us". I knew what he meant and it was a hard one to answer. At times like this I felt my heart was breaking. I talked with my daughter Pam about this, I felt so helpless. I needed her imput.

I really got nervous when they started using a machine to hoist him out of bed and into his wheel chair or into the bathroom. It just did not look steady enough to hold him. This was also the beginning of a long, long time of trying to get a wheel chair that was suitable for his height and weight. In fact right up to the end of his stay the wheel chair was not right.

Bob frequently had difficulty with food, he would eat some and then choke. This is one of the things that we were to expect.

So in March of 2002, Doctor Reginball told me that Bob would not last another year and he was going to put him on hospice if that was what I wanted. So I agreed to that with a heavy heart. This was so hard to even think about, it was hard to talk to the nurse I felt totally washed out right now. At the time I thought hospice would just be watching over Bob until he died, that it was really the end.

I discovered how wonderful Hospice is, they bathed him, gave him back rubs, saw to his medicines, saw that he had juice in the room at all times. In general they encouraged him.

I went to church and heard a fine message on calling on the Lord and laying all our cares on Him. I tried to begin to do that, because I can't call the shots, I just had to go along with what was going on with Bob and accept it. Give me courage dear Lord.

One day Bob kissed my hand, that made me happy. I held his hand a lot, he seemed to need that. He seemed to be responding to all the loving care the hospice group did for him. It seemed like he was getting better. The social worker talked to me on the way out one day and said, "Remember there are ups and downs in this, just enjoy the ups".

In April 2002 we began planning for Bob's passing. My daughter and I met with the pastor to discuss a memorial service. I also went to a lawyer to make sure all the paper work was in order. Then we had a funeral parlor person come and make arrangements for Bob to be cremated, per his desire. After I had that behind me, I needed to choose songs for the service. I still didn't feel Bob would die for a long while despite what every one else was saying.

At my next visit he would not even look at me. I needed to get used to the fact that he was no longer mine. He gets along good with all the personnel. I asked him if he liked the young girls taking care of him and he nodded his head. They all mention to me how well he responds to them and how he smiles at them. I felt hurt that he would respond to them and not me. He rarely smiled when I was with him. I would feed him and he would eat all of his meal with his eyes looking away from me. This was so hard on me. One day I was crying while I was there. He did not even notice this. I felt that we had him in a good place even though he would not respond to either Pam or me. I felt rejected and alone.

Another day he looked at me and squeezed my hand and that was enough for me. I just needed that encouragement.

One morning I went to church and heard a good sermon on contentment. I feel content and yet, I shouldn't feel that way. I think that when I decided to leave Bob in the nursing home I felt like I was laying down my burden and that now others would take care of him. It is so strange to think of him as a burden instead of a husband, lover, friend.

After church I went to Baskin Robbins and got two sundae's. By the time I got them back to Bob the whipped cream had all melted. But the ice cream was good and so was the fudge sauce. Bob really enjoyed it. He was much more responsive to me after that. He kissed me and answered somewhat when I would say something to him. He even smiled the smile I love. So hot fudge sundae's here I come.

I sold my house to my Grandson. On May 2002 I moved into Pam and Chuck's house into the basement apartment that they made for me. The church helped me move. It was quite an operation. The apartment was really lovely, just right for me.

One time Bob and I chatted for a while, but I could see that he was depressed. I saw a tear going down his face. I asked him how he felt and he said fine. Then I asked him how his heart felt and he said terrible. How could I blame him, it was a terrible situation to be in, and I knew he did not like it. However I still knew it was the best of places for him.

Bob went to some of the activities that they have for residents at the nursing home, especially if that included some music which he enjoys.

Mealtime always seemed to be difficult for Bob. The aides would feed him sometimes in his room if he was real tired. One day the aide that was feeding him thought he was all through. She left and I kept feeding him after the aide left and he ate a lot more for me. It was so nice to help feed him. He was wide awake through it all and responded to me somewhat. At least I understood what he wanted. I bent down and kissed his hand. He lifted my hand up to his mouth and kissed my hand. I was so very touched by that.

Bob seemed to be getting better with all the good work the hospice group was doing. I would read to him and share pictures with him and feed him on a regular basis. Seemed like I had less and less strength all the time. I needed to keep busier. However I would just fall asleep in his chair if I didn't have anything to do for him.

Bob seems to be responding to me and seemed interested in what I had to say. I think he is getting better. Pam would say watch out for a fall Mom. I don't believe that he only has six months to live. Hope breathes eternal in my soul I guess.

Every Sunday I would go to church and leave early so that I could get to the nursing home and feed Bob his dinner. We were allowed to eat in the chapel, it was small and very cozy for us. I would usually buy an extra lunch for myself so I would eat too, but I did not enjoy the meals very much, I was more interested in feeding him as much as I could. It made me feel less guilty to do this for him.

Hospice took him off one of his medicines, and that made a difference in his ability to speak plainer. He actually could get a few words out. It is wonderful to see the progress that he has made since Hospice has come in. I think he liked that extra attention that they gave to him.

I tried to keep his room as cheerful as possible. I always had blooming flowers in his window and pictures from home on the wall which I would change occasionally.

During the time Bob was confined at Heartwood I met several other women who were in the same boat as I was. We would compare notes with each other as to what was going on in the life of our husbands. Often it would come up with how we were feeling through all of this, and how we were reacting. All the ladies that I became acquainted with lost their husband before I did and I found out from them somewhat what to expect to happen near the end.

During Bob's stay I had a lot of contact with Medicare, it is a blessing to have Medicare, but it is a lot of work keeping up with the requirements. I had to keep in touch with them every month and account for any changes in my finances.

During this period of time most of my day's comprised of going to the nursing home and trying to wake Bob up sometimes to no avail and trying to feed him. The ups and downs were continual I never knew how he would respond to me in any day. Whether he would know me or reject me.

During the time of hospice I found that he was enjoying TV again, and we watched a lot of programs together which he seemed to enjoy. He seemed to be getting a new lease on life. In regards to food, at first Bob used weighted spoons and forks. Then he was on pureed food for a while, then soft food, then back to pureed food, then to mostly liquid. This seems to be in the progression of dementia and is to be expected. Regular food he chewed forever on and that made him tired, too tired to finish a meal.

I found out that even though I did not have the primary care of Bob, I still can be helpful to his healing I could stay alert to his physical pain and check with the nurses often as to what was being done for him. If he needed something I could make sure he got it. We don't have to completely give up all control or participation.

In August of 2002, I was able to bring Bob home for a visit. After that day I would bring him home for a three hour visit. He sometimes slept the whole time he was here other times we watched TV and I always tried to fix something that he might enjoy eating and could eat. It was always difficult though, because he was confined to his wheel chair. We were fortunate that the city transit would bring him right to the door and push him into the house and return and take him out to the bus later.

In August our whole family was gathering for a wedding and it was so nice that they all came to the nursing home to see Bob. We reserved one of the sun rooms and were able to all fit in there and have fellowship together. Bob was so pleased to see the whole family, so was I. He was glad to see kids and happy people but in reality he did not know who they were.

I joined the spouses group at Heartwood and it does help discussing what is going on in our lives. We met once a month, just a few ladies and sometimes a man. All of us are in the same boat. One day in particular I was talking with another wife who had just lost her husband to demensia. She was telling me through her tears that he had been dying for so long and that it makes it easier in the end.

In the nursing home if there is any infectious diseases going around they ask you to stay home. This happened a few times while Bob was confined there. This is a blessing to the patients, it keeps bad things from spreading.

As the years rolled by, I learned to just go along with Bob's hallucinating. If he asked something about a person who had died, I just went along with his thought. It is not wise to try and straighten him out at times like this. The reason for this is that you just can't straighten them out, their minds will not work the way ours does.

The main complaints that he had in the nursing home was about food, but that was because he could not chew his food properly or was just too tired to eat. At times he would tell me he did not have any breakfast or lunch, I checked and found out he had. This was due to his dementia of forgetting.

For our 61st wedding anniversary I bought a huge bouquet of flowers for the table in the chapel. Then I brought place mats from home and candles and set up a little anniversary dinner. We enjoyed being together that day. He did recognize me and he did try and talk a little. His answers usually were a yes or no or a nod of his head.

It was in September that the doctor took Bob off hospice. He was doing so much better, responding better and eating some better. I was glad that he got off hospice, but they were so good to him I think that is why he got some better.

From then on it was an on and off kind of relationship for us. I would visit him daily and do everything that I could for him. It was possible for me to keep track of his medication and what he ate. At times he would eat fairly well, but as the year progressed he got to a point where he was just too tired to eat. They fed him every day, but it was difficult even for the aides to have him eat all of his meals. They went from regular food, to soft food, to pureed food, to mostly liquid again.

As for me, I too was becoming more tired all the time. Often I would fall asleep holding his hand. Sometimes we had TV on and I would fall asleep soon after Bob did.

While Bob was a resident he fell from his bed. He seemed to be trying to get out of bed and go someplace. His legs were not strong enough to hold him, so he would fall. Sometimes he would fall from his walker. He constantly had an alarm system pinned to him so that if he fell it would go off. They even lowered his bed so he wouldn't fall so far.

One time only Bob called me on the phone. He got some help from the nurses to make the call, but he certainly wanted to talk to his wife. I was so pleased that he called, however, I did not know a word that he said except hello.

Bob was in a period where he could feed himself again, wanted to watch TV, wanted to go to church in the dining room. He seemed to be coming along just fine. If only he could have been able to walk I would have taken him home to live for a while.

Then he had a time where he was aggressive, showing poor behavior with one of the nurses and tried to get out a back door. His speech became more and more slurred and eventually he didn't try to talk anymore.

One morning I was listening to records and suddenly felt very sad. Thinking that I would never have Bob's arms around me to hug me. Never have him just want to love me, never have him really kiss me like he meant it. Never discuss affairs with him. Never be able to just talk to him without being concerned about how he would feel about whatever we talk about. It was a gloomy day and I felt gloomy too. Tears were coming too soon. I just want to cry and cry for no reason at all. I still remember that music. I think the songs were about no one like you. I lost my Bob a long time ago, in fact I can not remember how long ago it was. I miss him so much now.

For quite a while I went through periods of deep depression, tears and sadness seemed to be my room mates. Eventually I went to a Christian Counselor. I went to him for several weeks and he did help me to get better control of myself.

One day when I went to see Bob, he was already up and watching TV in the TV room. He was really enjoying the movie. I brought him the picture of us then and now for his room. He asked me after I kissed him, what are you doing here. So I said coming to see you. Since we were in the TV room and other people were there I did not do much communicating. One of the girls came in and told me on Halloween that he had children come into the room and he gave them candy and then asked them to open them up for him to eat. Then the aides told him he was supposed to give the candy to the children. So he said, "Why".

Around this time the physical therapy people got him to walk a half of a halls length with his walker. It was so good to see him on his feet.

He wanted to go outside. So one of the aids wheeled him outside and he enjoyed some fresh air. His main reason for wanting to go outside was so that he could get in the car and leave to go home. So when he got out there as soon as the girl left he said he wanted to get in the car. I said no way. Lord I don't know how to handle this, please make it plain to me how to go about this problem.

One of the girls from our Maranatha Children's Home in Alaska came by for a visit. We went to see Bob and he was just elated. I have never seen him so happy to see anyone. Catherine hugged him and she was so loving to him. He just loved it.

Every three months the staff would meet with my daughter and I to discuss Bob's condition. They would express any problems and so would my daughter and myself. It was a good time of catching up on Bob's physical condition. Also for getting things accomplished in his behalf.

For those of you who are going through this same process. Here are some of the things that I did with Bob at the nursing home. We most always read the Bible together. He was very receptive to that and two or three times he prayed out loud. I would read stories from the Reader's Digest and the Guideposts to him, some-times I would just tell him the stories, he could follow that better. We would often listen to music on his CD player, or look at the headlines in the newspaper. At times I would feed him and I usually brought him some Hershey bars which he loved. Sometimes I would push him around in his wheel chair, but this was difficult for me. We would attend some of the programs at the nursing home in the dining room. The staff did a great job of making the dining room look festive for the big holidays. I often held his hand until he went to sleep. These were the main things that we did together. In my heart I knew that often he didn't know who I was but I was there for him all the time.

I had lots of ideas of what we could do together. Like play some games, do some quizzes but none of that appealed to Bob. He was never a person who played games. I would have grand ideas about taking him out to meals in a restaurant. This idea he loved. I took him on off hours at a restaurant and we went to the quietest place available. He liked it, he never ate much, but the atmosphere was good for him. It tired him out a lot, so I was always glad when our transit ride came to take him back.

At times when I left his room feeling pretty blue, I would stop by one of the little ladies in another room and try and cheer her up. It worked for me too.

During Bob's stay I got him a recliner for his room. It made the room quite crowded but he did enjoy it when they put him in his chair, got his feet up and he rested comfortably so much better than in his wheelchair.

I took a volunteer job working in the gift shop at the nursing home. I worked there one day a week. It was nice because I could see Bob as they took him to physical therapy and to his meals. They were gracious enough to allow him to come into the shop. Sometimes, again, he would not know me. Other patients thought it was great I was there to sell them candy.

I got a cell phone so that I could be in contact with the nursing home at any time. We also used it to contact family members so Bob could talk to them. He never did much talking but he did enjoy hearing from other people. Especially he enjoyed talking to our son Paul. Two months after his last call with Paul my son died. My heart was broken to think I would never be able to talk or see my son Paul again on this earth. My only solace was that I would see him in heaven I was devastated and was not sure how to handle it with Bob. I was advised not to mention it. However, I did tell him because I thought he had a right to know. We both cried and clung to each other. After that he rarely mentioned Paul. He did not mention any of our other three children either for that matter. I would speak about them and tell him what was going on with them but it just did not register.

As for me I was overwhelmed with grief. I would go to the nursing home and the aides would offer sympathy and I would dissolve in tears. All down the hall to Bob's room I would be crying. When I got to his door, I would straighten up and try and get a smile on my face. I felt that I should be strong, and I knew that in God's word he gives us comfort however I just had a hard time being strong.

Our whole family came for the memorial service for Paul. When they came into the room we were in, I said to Bob, "Here is all your family". He said, "I don't know who these people are". That was a sad occasion for me.

At least Bob remembered his mother. He was very close to his mother as a child, so it is not surprising that he often mentioned her in the nursing home. He expected her to come and see him and in fact often thought he had just seen her in the hall. She seemed to be his favorite memory.

In retrospect I realize that Bob was so much better after he was released from Hospice. He would seem to try a little harder to do things, and to be a part of the people at the nursing home. As I go back over my notes I realize that during the years of 2003 and 2004 we had settled down into a routine kind of living. Visiting him, bringing him home for visits, taking him to restaurants, bringing him his favorite candy Hershey bars, and feeding him on Sunday noon meal.

Things went so well for him that I was not afraid to go to Alaska on a trip to visit our Children's Home location in Fairbanks. An opportunity came for me to go to Alaska with my daughter-in-law. I told Bob I was going to take this break for my health's sake. I got brave, and decided to take the break and go for a two weeks trip to Alaska. I needed to get completely away. I went to visit friends and to see Maranatha Children's Home's location. At the same time I was able to travel a bit around Alaska which I never got around to when we lived there. It was a good time of relaxation for me, and I came back refreshed.

A very lovely lady came in to visit Bob with her Alaskan husky dog, he enjoyed having the dog there and petting it. Her visits were something for him to look forward to when the nurses would tell him she was coming.

During Bob's last year, 2005, he began to go downhill. He had more episodes of hallucinations, more times of not knowing who I was.

Eventually the staff gave up on trying to make him walk a few steps. He was not strong enough for that. His swallowing began to be a big problem for him. His eating became such a problem that he had to be moved in with a group of people who had the same problem as him. This distressed me because he ate his meals looking at a wall in the dining room. This was necessary I was told, because he looked around the room instead of eating.

Bob was having more hallucinating, mostly about his mother, other times about fires or some other harmful thing. More times than not he did not recognize me. When he did I was happy. Other times I would just live with his dementia.

At one time his blood pressure was very low and he was losing weight again. The doctor took him off all medicine, I guess to give his body a break. At that time I was really glad for this verse from the "For, I am the Lord, your God, who takes hold of your right hand, and says to you, do not fear; I will help you". Isaish 41:13 It helped me to cope with what is going on.

My poor Bob he doesn't know where he is and questions this frequently. I can't believe how it must feel to not know where you are. At one time he asked me not to give up on him. One of his rational times. There were other rational times, often affected by the medicine he was taking. At one time they had him on predizone and suddenly this made him very talkative. He talked to everyone and preached when he was in his wheelchair in the hallway. He was preaching to young people, pressing them to get the Holy Spirit. I was walking down the hallway that particular day and I could hear him at quite a distance.

The nurses were all in awe that he would talk this much when for three years he hardly said anything to them. They had to take him off this medicine because it was affecting other parts of his body in the wrong way. After the medicine wore off he was back to his old self not talking to most people. He did mumble some to me but no conversation.

But, it had been nice to have conversations with him for that short period. I was warned continually that I should be prepared this would not last. This was true.

Gradually Bob started taking a longer time eating his meals, even if it was mostly liquid. He would usually be the last one out of the dining room at meal time. Sometimes when I fed him he would let the food dribble out of his mouth. Then he did this with anything he drank also.

In April of 2005, Bob started to get a rash on his legs. They treated him for this, but it got worse, much worse and he had to be taken to the dermatologist. She gave us prescriptions for medicine to be used on his body. After she got test results she found out it was MRSA, which is very contagious. After another two visits she said he also had Scabies, which is also very contagious. His whole body was covered with a bright red color and was itchy. His clothes would have blood on them because of the scratching. His body was just too weak to fight this infection that he had. By August he was just helpless with this terrible itch. The medicine was helping a little but not much, he needed extra care from everyone. I had to wear rubber gloves when I went in to visit him and wash my hands thoroughly when I was ready to leave.

I went down to the shore for a prayer retreat in August. While I was there I kept in contact with the nursing home. The last day I was there I talked to Bob's doctor and she informed me that he was losing weight too fast, and they could not get him to eat anything. Therefore she was suggesting that they put tubes into his body and feed him that way or call Hospice in. I questioned her at length the pro's and con's of this. I remembered how kind Hospice was and helpful. I also remembered that Bob did not want any undo help if he was dying. So with deep regret I said Hospice, because I knew that is what Bob wanted.

I rushed home to be with Bob. When I got to the hospital I discovered that when he was put on Hospice they took away all medicine and food and water. I was informed that any food or water he gagged on and would throw up and it would go down to his lungs and give him pneumonia. That would make him even more uncomfortable. That shocked me. I knew how good Hospice was before in taking care of his needs. However he was not on Hospice yet, they had not come in to see him. He was so thirsty, I took sponge swabs and moistened the inside of his mouth. I tried to keep his lips wet.

August 24, 2005, one sad day, it is hot, the fan is whirring away bringing in a little air. All the time Bob is awake he is uncomfortable. He moans and lifts his hands up to someone I can't see. He wants me to hold his hand, and then tires of that too weak to hold on. He lies with his mouth open sometimes shaking his head. Constantly seeming to try and readjust his night shirt and the sheet that is on him. Every once in a while scratching his itchy body, not as bad as before but still irritating him.

On and off I had my doubts about not having the tubes in his stomach so he could be fed. I looked for conformation on my decision. I felt like I was starving him to death, like I am guilty for all of this. How could I do this to Bob I promised to take care of him and here I was starving him, no food, no water, no medicines for the pain. My heart is breaking. That night I did a lot of crying.

On August 25th they put Bob on oxygen. He was having a lot of trouble breathing and the mask was bothering his face. His knees were turning color a nurse pointed out to me. This was a sign that something was shutting down, also his breathing was shutting down. I spent the afternoon singing hymns to him, especially the ones I knew that he loved.

The nurse recommended me to tell Bob that I would let him go. I realized several people had said that to me. So I got up real close and whispered to him that I would be all right if he leaves me, that he could go now. I told him how much I loved him, and that we will meet in heaven bye and bye.

I went home to eat, and my daughter Phyllis brought me an article on having the tube put into your stomach. It was very informative and I felt very very relieved, it sounded like a cruel thing to do to a person. I then felt that I had done the right thing, thank you Lord for a daughter who knows how to get the right information at the right time. This was the conformation that I needed and I accepted it as that.

Through the night I called the nursing home several times. I had been told that it could be a few hours or a month or so. On August 26th around 1AM, I received a call that Bob was gone. He went to a far better place. He was suffering so much that last day that I had asked the prayer chain at church to pray, "If it is God's will that Bob will be taken quickly". So I was both sad and content that Bob has met his maker.

My daughters Pam and Phyllis and I went right up to the nursing home to say our last goodbye's. He looked very peaceful for the first time in a long, long time. The nurses had folded his hands on his chest. It seemed to me that I could see him breathe. I could hear him breathe, but it turns out it was the man in the next bed. I kept putting my hands on his chest, because I was sure I saw it moving. His hands and arms were cold, I kissed him and tried to hug him one more time.

The songs that I sang to him yesterday ran through my mind. We had a good life together, a few days short of 64 years. Been many places together, done many things together and shared joys and laughter together.

But for the last ten years I have been losing Bob one way or another. God has been good to me to make this so gradual. It has been a long, long time since we slept together. A long time since we sat down at a meal together. A long time since he had shown me any affection. A long time since we had a conversation about anything. Now suddenly it is a short time since he has left this old earth.

To see the decline in my husband and to gradually lose all of our close relationships has been devastating. I feel like I really lost my husband years before he died. However, I found a deeper relationship with the Lord. Where I used to depend on my Bob for answers I now learned to depend on the Lord.

About the Author

Winifred E. Johnson was born on July 3, 1919 and raised in Yonkers, New York. She also lived in Pennsylvania, Alaska, Washington, Arizona, Oregon, New Jersey and California. Both her husband Bob, (who this story is about) and Winifred loved to travel. They went to Hawaii, England, Mexico, Canada and the Caribbean's as well as extensively in the United States.

She received a BA in Education in Flagstaff, AZ and a MA in education Seattle, WA.

Was a teacher in Bothell, WA, Port Angeles, WA, Cottonwood, AZ and Newhall, CA. Also a missionary in Fairbanks, AK and Cottonwood, AZ.

The hobbies that she enjoy were: crochet, ceramics, bead work, candle decorating and needle point. At the present time she spends time on the computer writing articles for magazines. She wrote and published a book called "Memories of Years Gone By" for her children.

Going to church is one ofthe important times of the week for her. At he present time she is living in Tacoma, WA with her daughter Pamella and son in law Chuck.

Writing this book was important to her because she wanted to reach out to other people who are going through the tough struggle with Alzheimer's.